Dedication

This book is dedicated to people who suffer from chronic wounds. It was written to encourage and empower you in your journey towards healing and recovery. As a wound care specialist, I am aware of your struggles and how life changing chronic wounds can be. There is hope. You are not alone.

To my dear friend, Maureen Jacobs, know that you are always in my prayers. Thank you for the gift of friendship.

Maria A Painter

He heals the Brokenhearted and Binds up their Wounds.

Psalm 147:3

This planner belongs to:

All things are possible

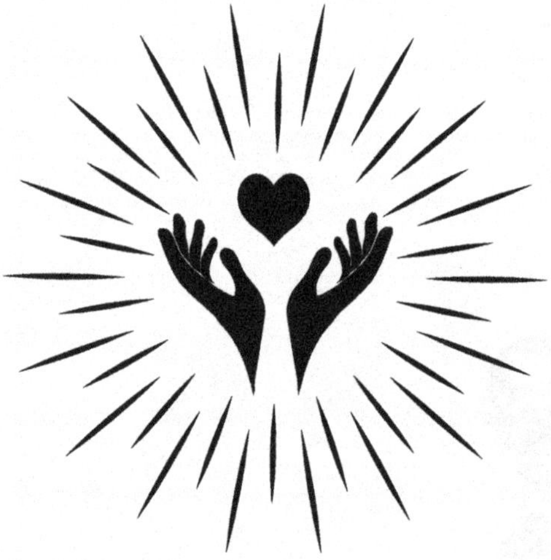

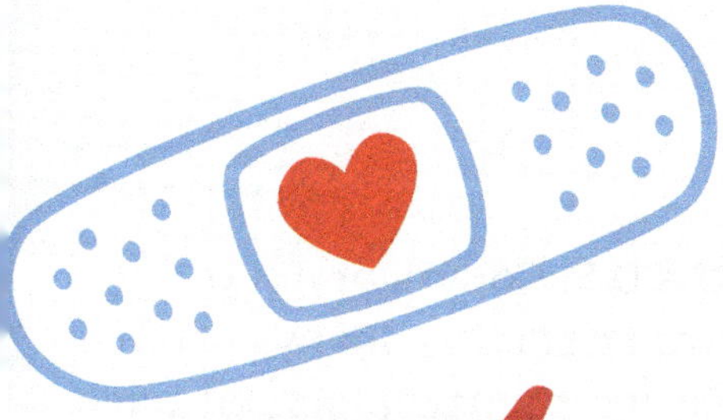

My Wound Healing Journey

MONTHLY PLANNER

Maria A Painter, BSND, DNP, AGNP, WSOC

Disclaimer: The recommendations in this book are general and may not be applicable to your specific needs and medical condition. Consult your doctor for specific guidelines for your care.

Maria A Painter, BSND, DNP, AGNP-BC, WSOC
Bachelor of Science in Nutrition/Dietetics, Doctor of Nursing Practice, Adult Geriatric Nurse Practitioner Board Certified, Wound, Skin, Ostomy Certified
Author, Illustrator, Cover Designer (elements used from CANVA)

ONLINE BOOKSTORE
http://touchtheheartreachthesoul.com

MERCHANDISE
http://touchtheheartreachthesoul.store

Featuring a collection of inspirational journals, notebooks, planners, art work and other gift items.

Disclaimer

The following clinical recommendations are based on 25 years of clinical experience working with patients from various clinical settings and best care practices. Each individual and case is different and requires an assessment and evaluation by a clinical provider. Consult with your doctor regarding your specific health care needs.

My desire is for you to become more involved in your wound care journey and make informed decisions. Wound care is complex and multifactorial therefore it is necessary to take an active approach and be fully committed in the process towards wound resolution and restoration of health.

Maria A Painter

GENERAL RECOMMENDATIONS

- ☐ Stay hydrated, choose low sugar beverages
- ☐ Eat more fresh fruits and vegetables
- ☐ Consider supplements to help with healing
- ☐ Increase consumption of lean meats
- ☐ Vitamins involved with healing: Vit A, C, D, E
- ☐ Get plenty of rest, most people need 8 hours
- ☐ Complete necessary diagnostic tests and labs
- ☐ Limit going to highly populated public spaces
- ☐ Stay up to date with your immunizations
- ☐ Stop smoking or cut back on smoking
- ☐ Stay active and walk; wear appropriate shoes
- ☐ If unable to walk, try chair exercises
- ☐ If bedbound: avoid pressure, try foam mattres
- ☐ If bedbound: change position every 1-2 hours
- ☐ Perform daily skin checks, in particular feet
- ☐ Keep bed linens clean and dry, change weekly
- ☐ Good hygiene and skin care are important
- ☐ Prayer & meditation can help relieve stress

GENERAL WOUND CARE RECOMMENDATIONS

- ☐ Keep the dressing clean and dry
- ☐ Change the dressing if visibly saturated
- ☐ Keep supplies at home to change the dressing
- ☐ Basic supplies: saline, gauze, pads, roll gauze
- ☐ Take your medications as instructed
- ☐ Follow up with doctor appointments
- ☐ Complete necessary diagnostic tests and labs
- ☐ Obtain medical devices: footwear, foot cover
- ☐ Be aware of signs & symptoms of infection
- ☐ Keep your work area and environment clean
- ☐ Monitor the size, appearance & drainage
- ☐ If you are diabetic, maintain control of sugar
- ☐ Keep pets away from area of wound(s)
- ☐ Protect wound(s) from injury, avoid falls
- ☐ Manage swelling with appropriate compression
- ☐ Compression is avoided in some cases
- ☐ Take an active role in your wound care
- ☐ Ask questions and stay informed

Consult your primary care doctor if you have questions.

WHEN TO SEEK URGENT CARE /NOTIFY DOCTOR

- ☐ Seek urgent care for the following conditions:
- ☐ Recognize when there is a change in wound(s)
- ☐ Infection: increased redness, swelling, pain
- ☐ Infection: yellow/green, thick drainage
- ☐ Severe infection: fever, chills, redness spreads
- ☐ Increased pain no longer controlled by OTC meds
- ☐ Recent fall or injury to affected side
- ☐ Diabetics: poorly controlled blood sugar
- ☐ Formation of a new wound, blister or rash
- ☐ Feeling sad, hopeless or depressed
- ☐ Decreased mobility, cannot care for yourself
- ☐ Change in support system (spouse in hospital)
- ☐ Transportation is not available
- ☐ Excessive bleeding from wound
- ☐ Change in wound appearance: has turned blac
- ☐ Loss of feeling/ numbness on affected extremity
- ☐ Unsafe home living environment
- ☐ When in doubt, call your primary care doctor

JANUARY

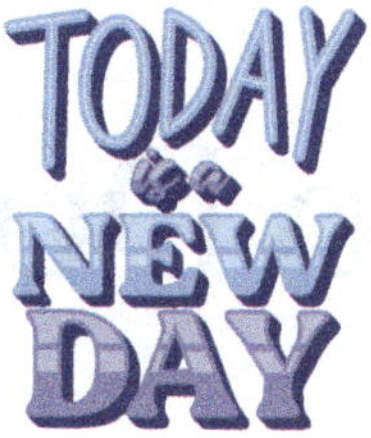

MONTH ____________________

MON	TUE	WED	THU	FRI	SAT	SUN

TO DO

- [ ]
- [ ]
- [ ]
- [ ]
- [ ]
- [ ]
- [ ]
- [ ]
- [ ]
- [ ]

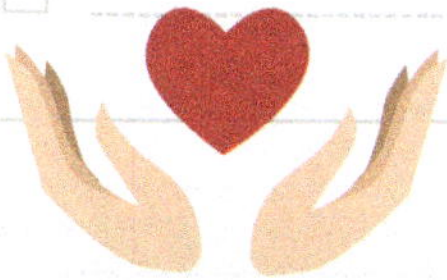

GOALS

- [ ]
- [ ]
- [ ]
- [ ]

NOTES

To Do List

NEVER give up!

Date : ....

- [ ]
- [ ]
- [ ]
- [ ]
- [ ]
- [ ]
- [ ]
- [ ]
- [ ]
- [ ]
- [ ]
- [ ]
- [ ]
- [ ]
- [ ]
- [ ]
- [ ]
- [ ]
- [ ]
- [ ]
- [ ]
- [ ]
- [ ]
- [ ]
- [ ]
- [ ]

NOTE :

Wound #1:

DATE:

WOUND CARE INSTRUCTIONS	NOTES

MEASUREMENTS (LENGTH X WIDTH X DEPTH) CM
COLOR OF WOUND, AMT OF DRAINAGE

Wound #2

DATE:

WOUND CARE INSTRUCTIONS	NOTES

MEASUREMENTS (LENGTH X WIDTH X DEPTH) CM
COLOR OF WOUND, AMT OF DRAINAGE

MEDICATION LIST

NAME:

DOCTOR:

medication	dose	frequency	time	notes

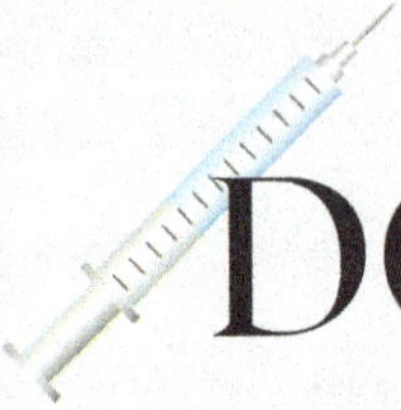

DOCTOR NOTES

DATE : ______________________ DOCTOR: ______________________

LOCATION: ______________________

DISCUSSION :

NOTES :

TO DO:

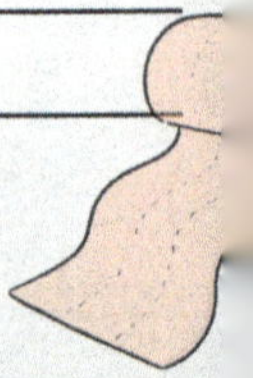

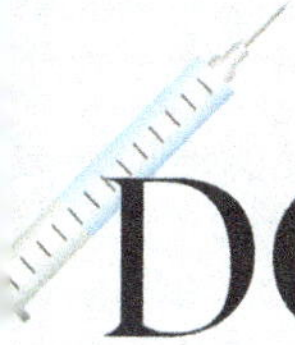

DOCTOR NOTES

DATE : ____________________ DOCTOR: ____________________

LOCATION: ____________________

DISCUSSION :

NOTES :

TO DO:

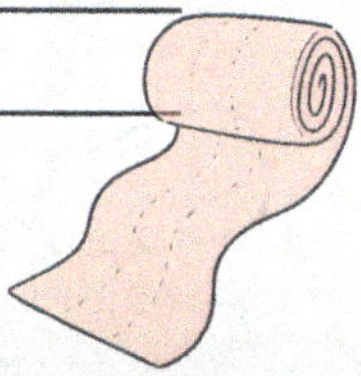

FEBRUARY

NEVER GIVE UP

MON	TUE	WED	THU	FRI	SAT	SUN

TO DO

- [ ]
- [ ]
- [ ]
- [ ]
- [ ]
- [ ]
- [ ]
- [ ]
- [ ]
- [ ]

GOALS

- [ ]
- [ ]
- [ ]
- [ ]

NOTES

To Do List

YOU GOT THIS!

Date : ....

- [ ] ____
- [ ] ____
- [ ] ____
- [ ] ____
- [ ] ____
- [ ] ____
- [ ] ____
- [ ] ____
- [ ] ____
- [ ] ____
- [ ] ____
- [ ] ____
- [ ] ____
- [ ] ____
- [ ] ____
- [ ] ____
- [ ] ____
- [ ] ____
- [ ] ____
- [ ] ____
- [ ] ____
- [ ] ____
- [ ] ____
- [ ] ____
- [ ] ____
- [ ] ____

NOTE :

Wound #1:

DATE:

WOUND CARE INSTRUCTIONS	NOTES

MEASUREMENTS (LENGTH X WIDTH X DEPTH) CM

COLOR OF WOUND, AMT OF DRAINAGE

Wound #2

DATE:

WOUND CARE INSTRUCTIONS	NOTES

MEASUREMENTS (LENGTH X WIDTH X DEPTH) CM
COLOR OF WOUND, AMT OF DRAINAGE

MEDICATION LIST

NAME: DOCTOR:

medication	dose	frequency	time	notes

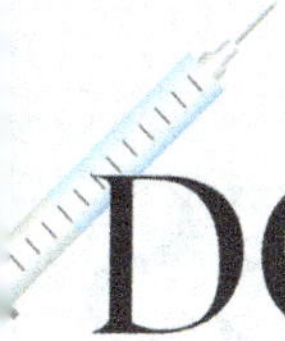

DOCTOR NOTES

DATE : ____________________ DOCTOR: ____________________

LOCATION: ____________________

DISCUSSION :

NOTES :

TO DO:

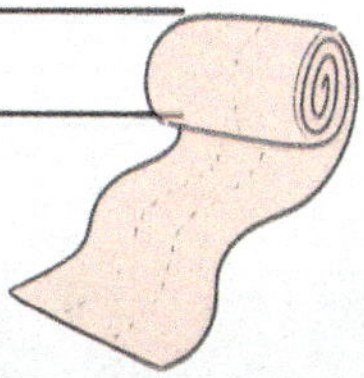

DOCTOR NOTES

DATE : ____________________ DOCTOR: ____________________

LOCATION: ____________________

DISCUSSION :

NOTES :

TO DO:

YOU ARE CAPABLE

MARCH

MONTH ....

MON	TUE	WED	THU	FRI	SAT	SUN

TO DO

- [ ]
- [ ]
- [ ]
- [ ]
- [ ]
- [ ]
- [ ]
- [ ]
- [ ]
- [ ]

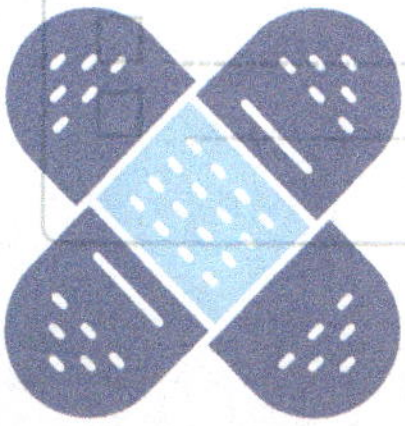

GOALS

- [ ]
- [ ]
- [ ]
- [ ]

NOTES

To Do List

enjoy every moment.

Date : ....

- [ ]
- [ ]

NOTE :

Wound #1:

DATE:

WOUND CARE INSTRUCTIONS	NOTES

MEASUREMENTS (LENGTH X WIDTH X DEPTH) CM

COLOR OF WOUND, AMT OF DRAINAGE

Wound #2

DATE:

WOUND CARE INSTRUCTIONS	NOTES

MEASUREMENTS (LENGTH X WIDTH X DEPTH) CM
COLOR OF WOUND, AMT OF DRAINAGE

MEDICATION LIST

NAME: DOCTOR:

medication	dose	frequency	time	notes

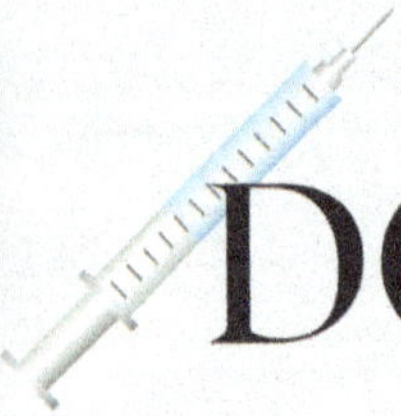

DOCTOR NOTES

DATE : ____________________ DOCTOR: ____________________

LOCATION: ____________________

DISCUSSION :

NOTES :

TO DO:

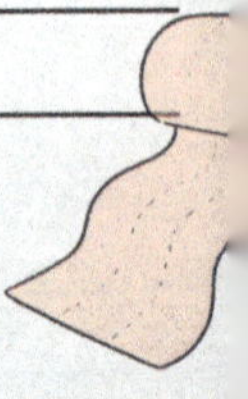

DOCTOR NOTES

DATE : ______________________ DOCTOR: ______________________

LOCATION: ______________________

DISCUSSION :

NOTES :

TO DO:

small step
everyday

APRIL

MONTH ____________________

MON	TUE	WED	THU	FRI	SAT	SUN

TO DO

- [ ] ____________________
- [ ] ____________________
- [ ] ____________________
- [ ] ____________________
- [ ] ____________________
- [ ] ____________________
- [ ] ____________________
- [ ] ____________________
- [ ] ____________________
- [ ] ____________________

GOALS

- [ ] ____________________
- [ ] ____________________
- [ ] ____________________
- [ ] ____________________

NOTES

To Do List

YOU ARE CAPABLE

Date : ....

NOTE :

Wound #1:

DATE:

WOUND CARE INSTRUCTIONS	NOTES

MEASUREMENTS (LENGTH X WIDTH X DEPTH) CM
COLOR OF WOUND, AMT OF DRAINAGE

Wound #2

DATE:

WOUND CARE INSTRUCTIONS	NOTES

MEASUREMENTS (LENGTH X WIDTH X DEPTH) CM
COLOR OF WOUND, AMT OF DRAINAGE

MEDICATION LIST

NAME:

DOCTOR:

medication	dose	frequency	time	notes

DOCTOR NOTES

DATE : ____________ DOCTOR: ____________

LOCATION: ____________

DISCUSSION :

NOTES :

TO DO:

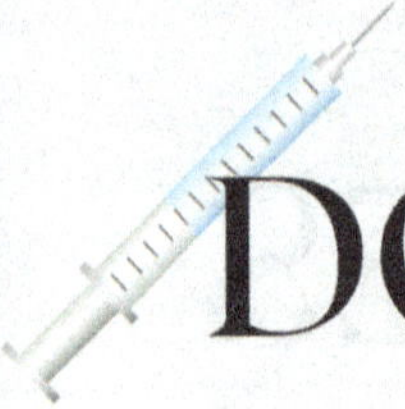

DOCTOR NOTES

DATE : DOCTOR:

LOCATION:

DISCUSSION : NOTES :

TO DO:

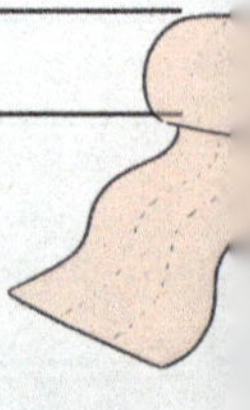

MAY

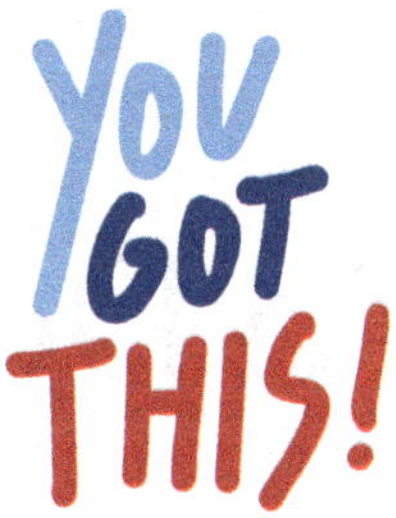

MON	TUE	WED	THU	FRI	SAT	SUN

TO DO

- [ ]
- [ ]
- [ ]
- [ ]
- [ ]
- [ ]
- [ ]

GOALS

- [ ]
- [ ]
- [ ]
- [ ]

NOTES

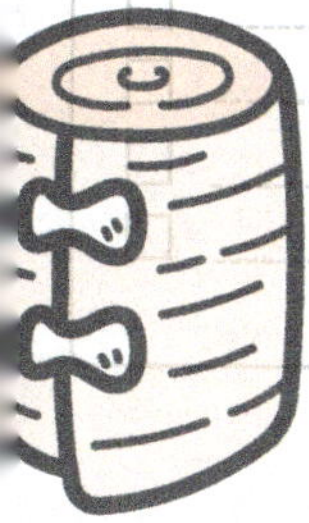

To Do List

small step everyday

Date : ....

NOTE :

Wound #1: ____________

DATE:

WOUND CARE INSTRUCTIONS	NOTES
✧	✧
✧	✧
✧	✧

MEASUREMENTS (LENGTH X WIDTH X DEPTH) CM
COLOR OF WOUND, AMT OF DRAINAGE

Wound #2

DATE:

WOUND CARE INSTRUCTIONS	NOTES

MEASUREMENTS (LENGTH X WIDTH X DEPTH) CM
COLOR OF WOUND, AMT OF DRAINAGE

MEDICATION LIST

NAME: DOCTOR:

medication	dose	frequency	time	notes

DOCTOR NOTES

DATE : ______________________ DOCTOR: ______________________

LOCATION: ______________________

DISCUSSION :

NOTES :

TO DO:

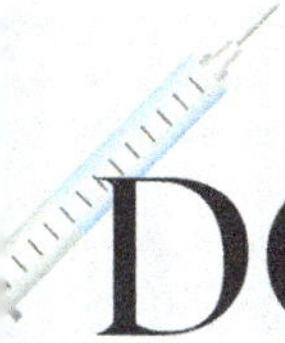

DOCTOR NOTES

DATE : ____________________ DOCTOR: ____________________

LOCATION: ____________________

DISCUSSION :

NOTES :

TO DO:

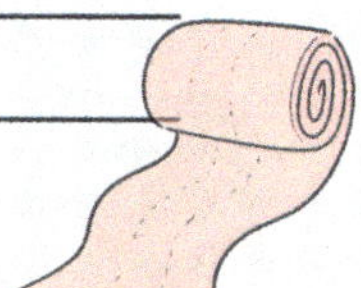

you can do it!

JUNE

MON	TUE	WED	THU	FRI	SAT	SUN

TO DO

- [ ]
- [ ]
- [ ]
- [ ]
- [ ]
- [ ]
- [ ]
- [ ]
- [ ]
- [ ]

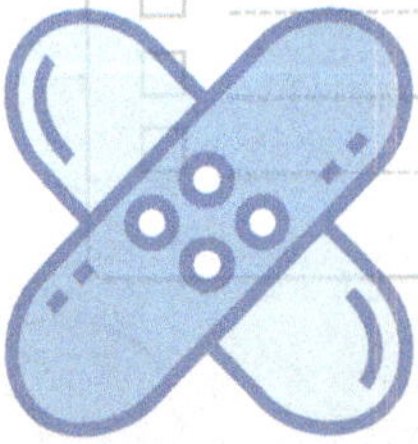

GOALS

- [ ]
- [ ]
- [ ]
- [ ]

NOTES

To Do List

Date : ....

smile each day

NOTE :

Wound #1: ____________________

DATE:

WOUND CARE INSTRUCTIONS	NOTES
✦	✦
✦	✦
✦	✦

MEASUREMENTS (LENGTH X WIDTH X DEPTH) CM
COLOR OF WOUND, AMT OF DRAINAGE

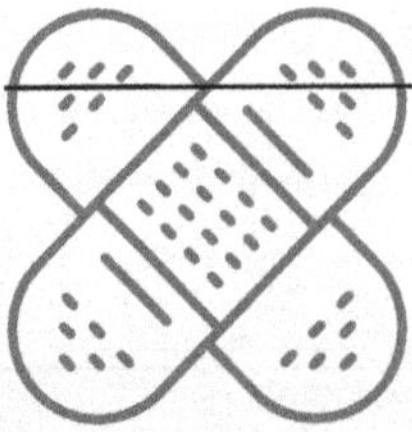

Wound #2

DATE:

WOUND CARE INSTRUCTIONS	NOTES

MEASUREMENTS (LENGTH X WIDTH X DEPTH) CM
COLOR OF WOUND, AMT OF DRAINAGE

MEDICATION LIST

NAME: ______________________ DOCTOR: ______________________

medication	dose	frequency	time	notes

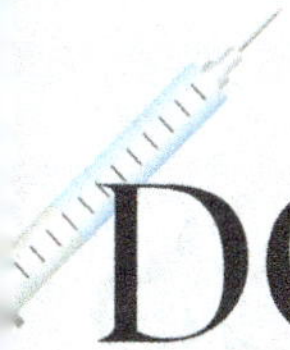

DOCTOR NOTES

DATE :

DOCTOR:

LOCATION:

DISCUSSION :

NOTES :

TO DO:

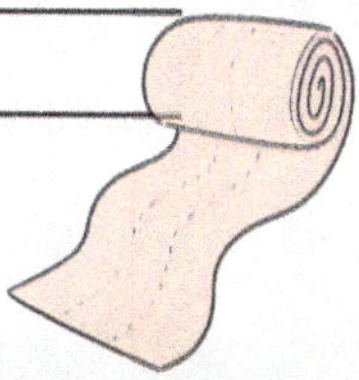

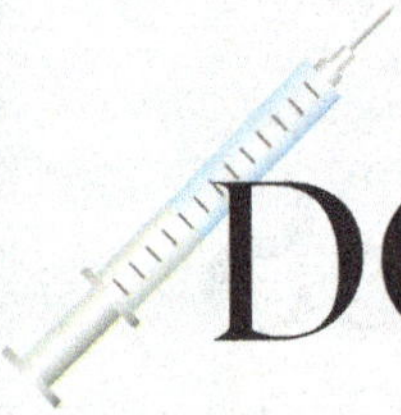

DOCTOR NOTES

DATE : ____________________ DOCTOR: ____________________

LOCATION: ____________________

DISCUSSION :

NOTES :

TO DO:

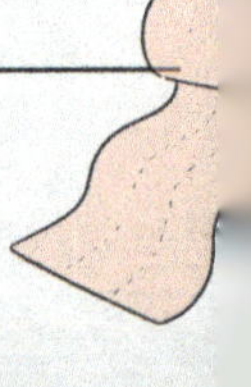

AUGUST

STAY STRONG!

MON	TUE	WED	THU	FRI	SAT	SUN

TO DO

GOALS

NOTES

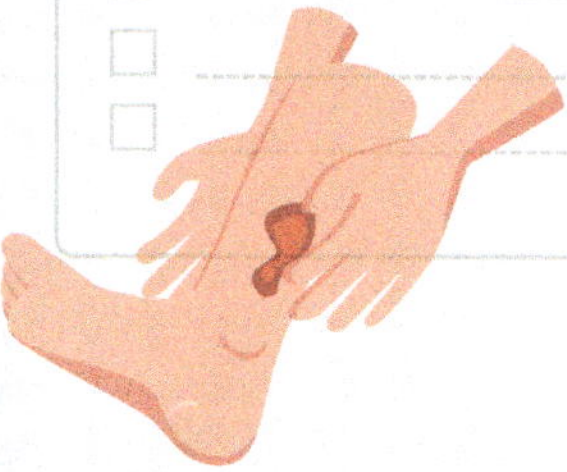

To Do List

breathe

Date : ....

- [ ] ____________________
- [ ] ____________________
- [ ] ____________________
- [ ] ____________________
- [ ] ____________________
- [ ] ____________________
- [ ] ____________________
- [ ] ____________________
- [ ] ____________________
- [ ] ____________________
- [ ] ____________________
- [ ] ____________________
- [ ] ____________________
- [ ] ____________________
- [ ] ____________________
- [ ] ____________________
- [ ] ____________________
- [ ] ____________________
- [ ] ____________________
- [ ] ____________________
- [ ] ____________________
- [ ] ____________________
- [ ] ____________________
- [ ] ____________________
- [ ] ____________________
- [ ] ____________________

NOTE :

Wound #1:

DATE:

WOUND CARE INSTRUCTIONS	NOTES

MEASUREMENTS (LENGTH X WIDTH X DEPTH) CM

COLOR OF WOUND, AMT OF DRAINAGE

Wound #2

DATE:

WOUND CARE INSTRUCTIONS	NOTES

MEASUREMENTS (LENGTH X WIDTH X DEPTH) CM

COLOR OF WOUND, AMT OF DRAINAGE

MEDICATION LIST

NAME:

DOCTOR:

medication	dose	frequency	time	notes

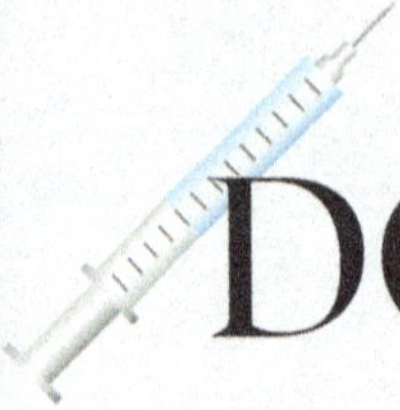

DOCTOR NOTES

DATE : ____________________ DOCTOR: ____________________

LOCATION: ____________________

DISCUSSION :

NOTES :

TO DO:

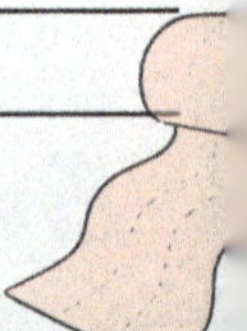

DOCTOR NOTES

DATE : ______________________ DOCTOR: ______________________

LOCATION: ______________________

DISCUSSION :

NOTES :

TO DO:

AUGUST

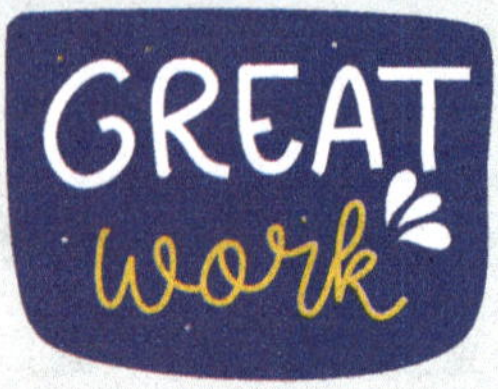

MON	TUE	WED	THU	FRI	SAT	SUN

TO DO

- [ ]
- [ ]
- [ ]
- [ ]
- [ ]
- [ ]
- [ ]
- [ ]
- [ ]
- [ ]

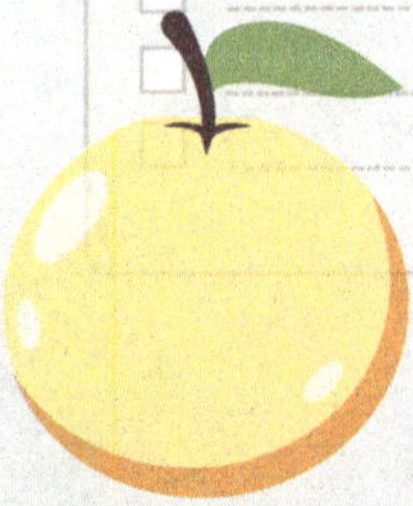

GOALS

- [ ]
- [ ]
- [ ]
- [ ]

NOTES

To Do List

Be proud of your self

Date : ....

NOTE :

Wound #1:

DATE:

WOUND CARE INSTRUCTIONS	NOTES

MEASUREMENTS (LENGTH X WIDTH X DEPTH) CM
COLOR OF WOUND, AMT OF DRAINAGE

Wound #2

DATE:

WOUND CARE INSTRUCTIONS	NOTES

MEASUREMENTS (LENGTH X WIDTH X DEPTH) CM
COLOR OF WOUND, AMT OF DRAINAGE

MEDICATION LIST

NAME: DOCTOR:

medication	dose	frequency	time	notes

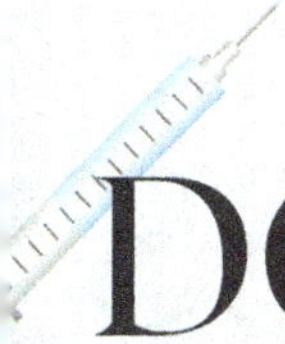

DOCTOR NOTES

DATE: ____________________ DOCTOR: ____________________

LOCATION: ____________________

DISCUSSION:

NOTES:

TO DO:

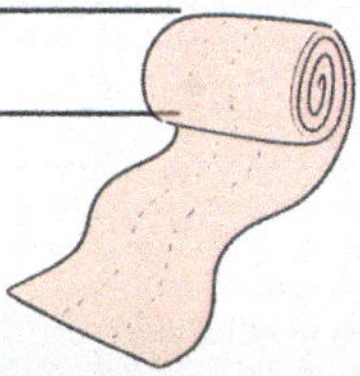

DOCTOR NOTES

DATE : ______________________ DOCTOR: ______________________

LOCATION: ______________________

DISCUSSION :

NOTES :

TO DO:

SEPTEMBER

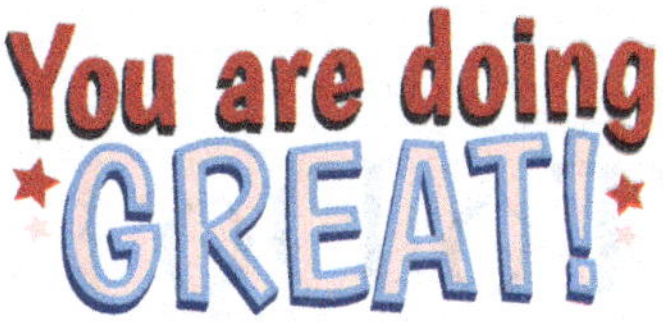

MON	TUE	WED	THU	FRI	SAT	SUN

TO DO

- [ ]
- [ ]
- [ ]
- [ ]
- [ ]
- [ ]
- [ ]
- [ ]
- [ ]
- [ ]

GOALS

- [ ]
- [ ]
- [ ]
- [ ]

NOTES

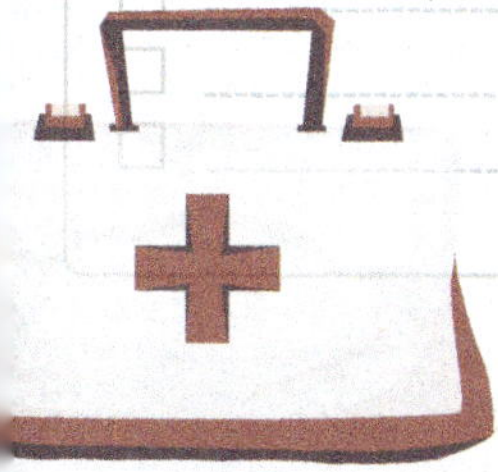

To Do List

always Think Positive

Date : ....

- [ ] ____________________
- [ ] ____________________
- [ ] ____________________
- [ ] ____________________
- [ ] ____________________
- [ ] ____________________
- [ ] ____________________
- [ ] ____________________
- [ ] ____________________
- [ ] ____________________
- [ ] ____________________
- [ ] ____________________
- [ ] ____________________
- [ ] ____________________
- [ ] ____________________
- [ ] ____________________
- [ ] ____________________
- [ ] ____________________
- [ ] ____________________
- [ ] ____________________
- [ ] ____________________
- [ ] ____________________
- [ ] ____________________
- [ ] ____________________
- [ ] ____________________
- [ ] ____________________

NOTE :

Wound #1:

DATE:

WOUND CARE INSTRUCTIONS	NOTES

MEASUREMENTS (LENGTH X WIDTH X DEPTH) CM
COLOR OF WOUND, AMT OF DRAINAGE

Wound #2

DATE:

WOUND CARE INSTRUCTIONS	NOTES

MEASUREMENTS (LENGTH X WIDTH X DEPTH) CM
COLOR OF WOUND, AMT OF DRAINAGE

MEDICATION LIST

NAME: DOCTOR:

medication	dose	frequency	time	notes

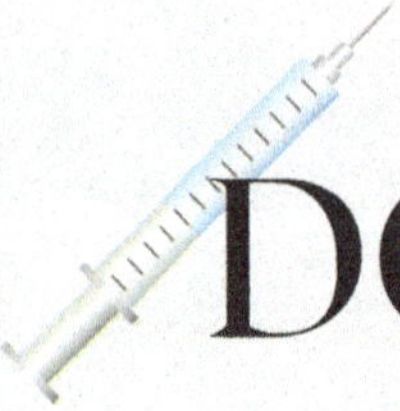

DOCTOR NOTES

DATE :

DOCTOR:

LOCATION:

DISCUSSION :

NOTES :

TO DO:

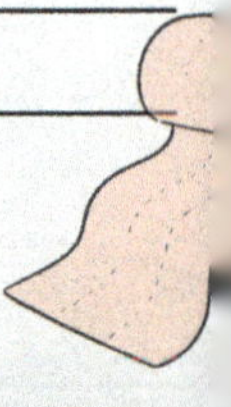

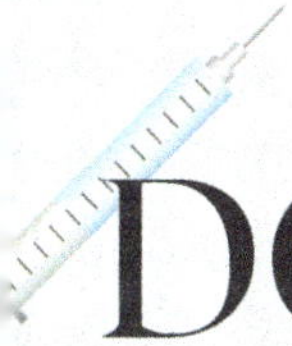

DOCTOR NOTES

DATE : ______________________ DOCTOR: ______________________

LOCATION: ______________________

DISCUSSION :

NOTES :

TO DO:

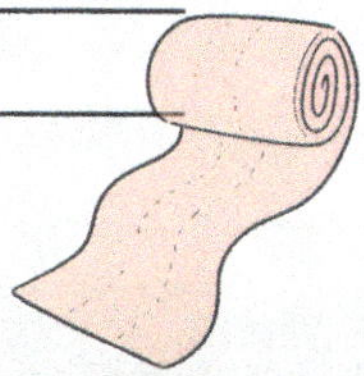

OCTOBER

YOU CAN DO IT!

MON	TUE	WED	THU	FRI	SAT	SUN

TO DO

- [ ]
- [ ]
- [ ]
- [ ]
- [ ]
- [ ]
- [ ]
- [ ]
- [ ]
- [ ]

GOALS

- [ ]
- [ ]
- [ ]
- [ ]

NOTES

To Do List

Don't Forget To Relax

Date : ....

- [ ] ______________________
- [ ] ______________________
- [ ] ______________________
- [ ] ______________________
- [ ] ______________________
- [ ] ______________________
- [ ] ______________________
- [ ] ______________________
- [ ] ______________________
- [ ] ______________________
- [ ] ______________________
- [ ] ______________________
- [ ] ______________________
- [ ] ______________________
- [ ] ______________________
- [ ] ______________________
- [ ] ______________________
- [ ] ______________________
- [ ] ______________________
- [ ] ______________________
- [ ] ______________________
- [ ] ______________________
- [ ] ______________________
- [ ] ______________________
- [ ] ______________________
- [ ] ______________________

NOTE :

Wound #1:

DATE:

WOUND CARE INSTRUCTIONS	NOTES

MEASUREMENTS (LENGTH X WIDTH X DEPTH) CM
COLOR OF WOUND, AMT OF DRAINAGE

Wound #2

DATE:

WOUND CARE INSTRUCTIONS	NOTES

MEASUREMENTS (LENGTH X WIDTH X DEPTH) CM
COLOR OF WOUND, AMT OF DRAINAGE

MEDICATION LIST

NAME: DOCTOR:

medication	dose	frequency	time	notes

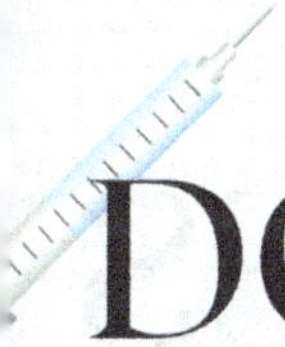

DOCTOR NOTES

DATE : ____________________ DOCTOR: ____________________

LOCATION: ____________________

DISCUSSION :

NOTES :

TO DO:

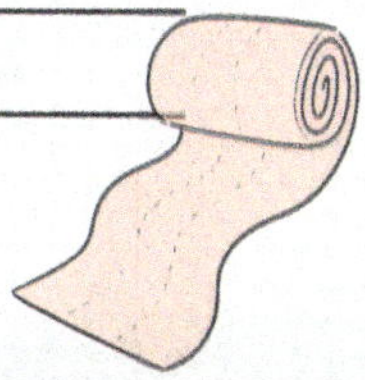

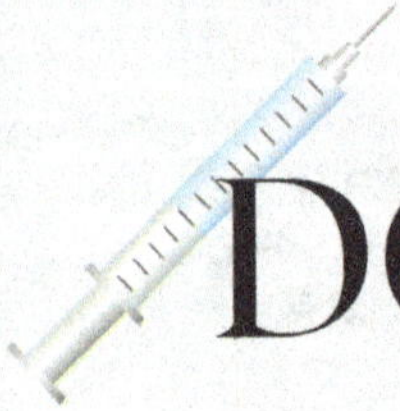

DOCTOR NOTES

DATE : ______________________ DOCTOR: ______________________

LOCATION: ______________________

DISCUSSION :

NOTES :

TO DO:

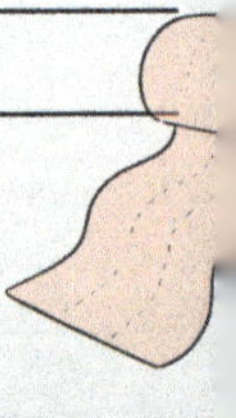

NOVEMBER

KEEP ON GOING

MON	TUE	WED	THU	FRI	SAT	SUN

TO DO

- [ ]
- [ ]
- [ ]
- [ ]
- [ ]
- [ ]
- [ ]
- [ ]
- [ ]
- [ ]

GOALS

- [ ]
- [ ]
- [ ]
- [ ]

NOTES

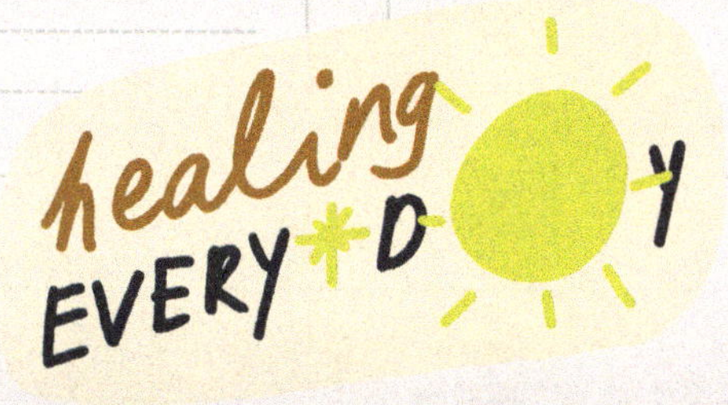

To Do List

Choose JOY

Date : ....

NOTE :

Wound #1:

DATE:

WOUND CARE INSTRUCTIONS	NOTES

MEASUREMENTS (LENGTH X WIDTH X DEPTH) CM
COLOR OF WOUND, AMT OF DRAINAGE

Wound #2

DATE:

WOUND CARE INSTRUCTIONS	NOTES

MEASUREMENTS (LENGTH X WIDTH X DEPTH) CM
COLOR OF WOUND, AMT OF DRAINAGE

MEDICATION LIST

NAME: ______________________ DOCTOR: ______________________

medication	dose	frequency	time	notes

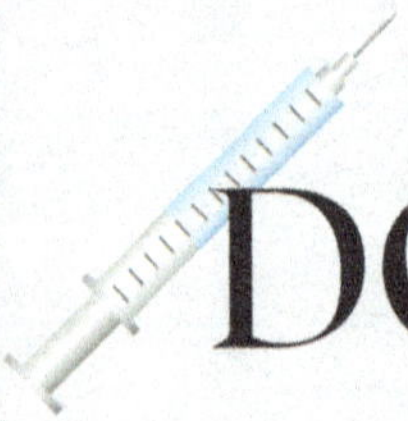

DOCTOR NOTES

DATE : ______________________ DOCTOR: ______________________

LOCATION: ______________________

DISCUSSION :

____
____
____
____
____
____
____
____
____

NOTES :

____
____
____
____
____
____
____
____
____

TO DO:

______________________ ______________________
______________________ ______________________
______________________ ______________________
______________________ ______________________
______________________ ______________________
______________________ ______________________
______________________ ______________________
______________________ ______________________

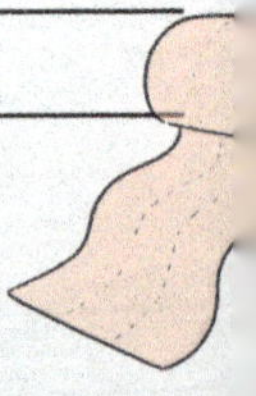

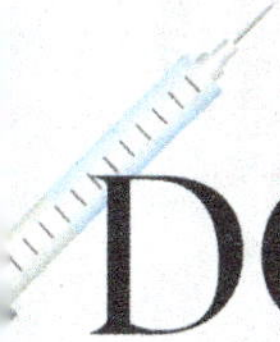

DOCTOR NOTES

DATE : ______________________ DOCTOR: ______________________

LOCATION: ______________________________

DISCUSSION :

NOTES :

TO DO:

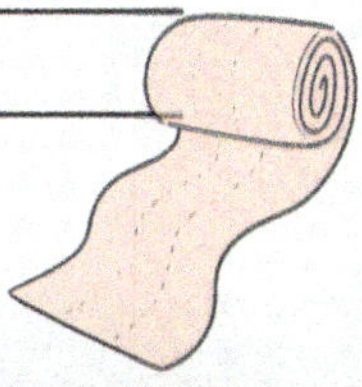

GOOD JOB

DECEMBER

MON	TUE	WED	THU	FRI	SAT	SUN

TO DO

- [ ]
- [ ]
- [ ]
- [ ]
- [ ]
- [ ]
- [ ]
- [ ]
- [ ]
- [ ]

GOALS

- [ ]
- [ ]
- [ ]
- [ ]

NOTES

HEAL TOGETHER

To Do List

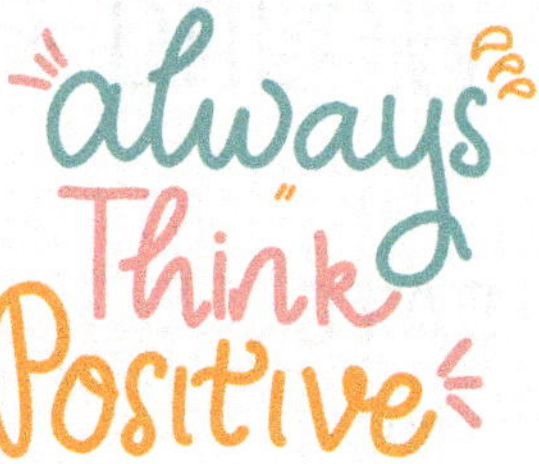

Date : ....

- [ ] ____________________ - [ ] ____________________
- [ ] ____________________ - [ ] ____________________
- [ ] ____________________ - [ ] ____________________
- [ ] ____________________ - [ ] ____________________
- [ ] ____________________ - [ ] ____________________
- [ ] ____________________ - [ ] ____________________
- [ ] ____________________ - [ ] ____________________
- [ ] ____________________ - [ ] ____________________
- [ ] ____________________ - [ ] ____________________
- [ ] ____________________ - [ ] ____________________
- [ ] ____________________ - [ ] ____________________
- [ ] ____________________ - [ ] ____________________
- [ ] ____________________ - [ ] ____________________

NOTE :

Wound #1:

DATE:

WOUND CARE INSTRUCTIONS	NOTES
✦	✦
✦	✦
✦	✦

MEASUREMENTS (LENGTH X WIDTH X DEPTH) CM
COLOR OF WOUND, AMT OF DRAINAGE

Wound #2

DATE:

WOUND CARE INSTRUCTIONS	NOTES

MEASUREMENTS (LENGTH X WIDTH X DEPTH) CM
COLOR OF WOUND, AMT OF DRAINAGE

MEDICATION LIST

NAME:

DOCTOR:

medication	dose	frequency	time	notes

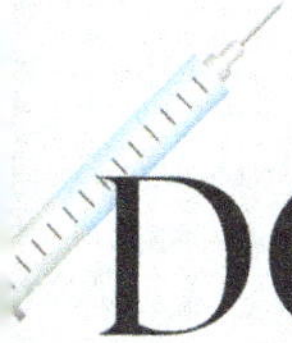

DOCTOR NOTES

DATE : ____________________ DOCTOR: ____________________

LOCATION: ____________________

DISCUSSION :

NOTES :

TO DO:

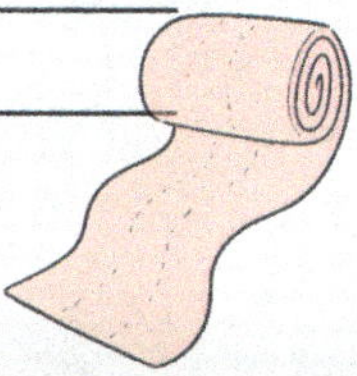

DOCTOR NOTES

DATE : ______________ DOCTOR: ______________

LOCATION: ______________

DISCUSSION :

NOTES :

TO DO:

ANTIBIOTIC LOG

NAME:

DOCTOR:

medication	dose	frequency	time	notes

ANTIBIOTIC LOG

NAME:

DOCTOR:

medication	dose	frequency	time	notes

ANTIBIOTIC LOG

NAME: ______________________ DOCTOR: ______________________

medication	dose	frequency	time	notes

PRIMARY CARE DOCTOR

NAME :
CONTACT :
ADDRESS :

EMAIL :
NOTES :

QUESTIONS FOR THE DOCTOR:

APPOINTMENTS:

TO DO:

CARDIOLOGIST

NAME :
CONTACT :
ADDRESS :

EMAIL :
NOTES :

QUESTIONS FOR THE DOCTOR:

APPOINTMENTS:

TO DO:

VASCULAR SURGEON

NAME :
CONTACT :
ADDRESS :

EMAIL :
NOTES :

QUESTIONS FOR THE DOCTOR:

APPOINTMENTS:

TO DO:

SURGEON

NAME :
CONTACT :
ADDRESS :

EMAIL :
NOTES :

QUESTIONS FOR THE DOCTOR:

APPOINTMENTS:

TO DO:

NUTRITIONIST

NAME :
CONTACT :
ADDRESS :

EMAIL :
NOTES :

QUESTIONS FOR THE DOCTOR:

APPOINTMENTS:

TO DO:

PODIATRIST

NAME :
CONTACT :
ADDRESS :

EMAIL :
NOTES :

QUESTIONS FOR THE DOCTOR:

APPOINTMENTS:

TO DO:

SPECIALIST

NAME :
CONTACT :
ADDRESS :

EMAIL :
NOTES :

QUESTIONS FOR THE DOCTOR:

APPOINTMENTS:

TO DO:

SPECIALIST

NAME :
CONTACT :
ADDRESS :

EMAIL :
NOTES :

QUESTIONS FOR THE DOCTOR:

APPOINTMENTS:

TO DO:

SPECIALIST

NAME :
CONTACT :
ADDRESS :

EMAIL :
NOTES :

QUESTIONS FOR THE DOCTOR:

APPOINTMENTS:

TO DO:

NOTES

date ____ / ____

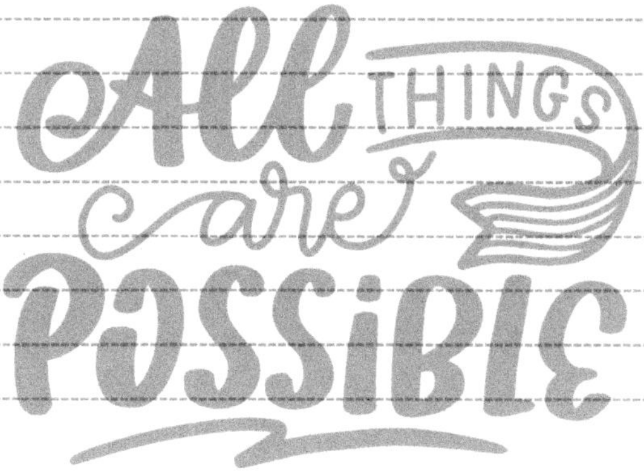

NOTES

date ____ / ____

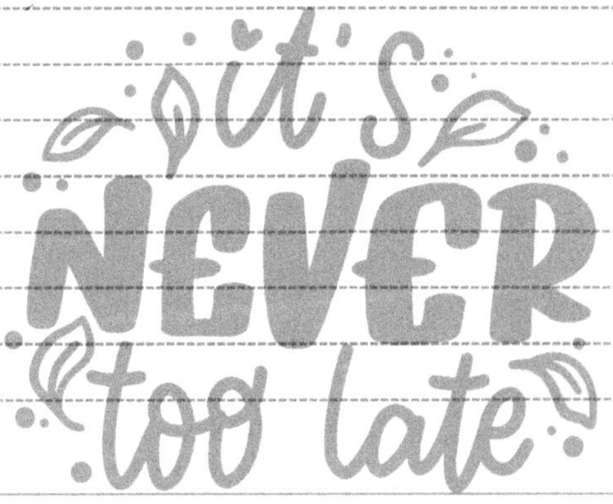

NOTES

date ____ / ____

trust your

JOURNEY

NOTES

date ___ / ___

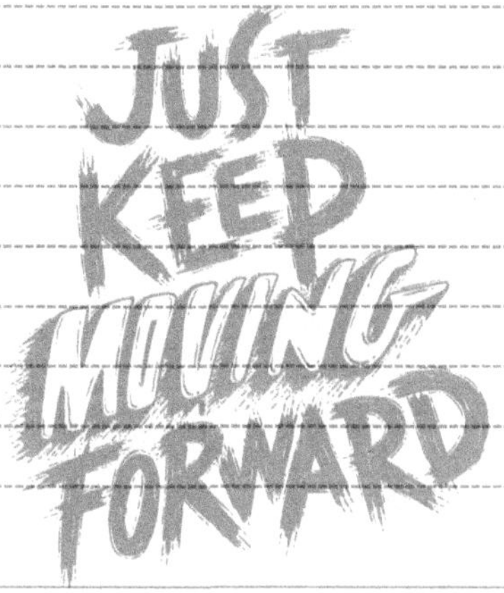

NOTES

date ____ / ____

Keep it up

NOTES

date ____ / ____

Happiness is a Choice

NOTES date ___ / ___

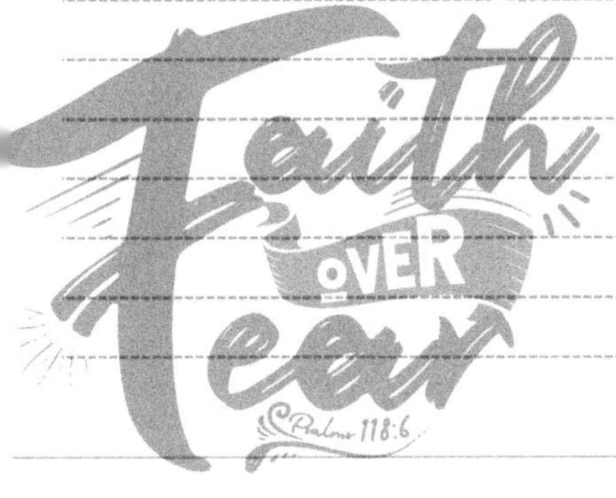

NOTES

date ____/____

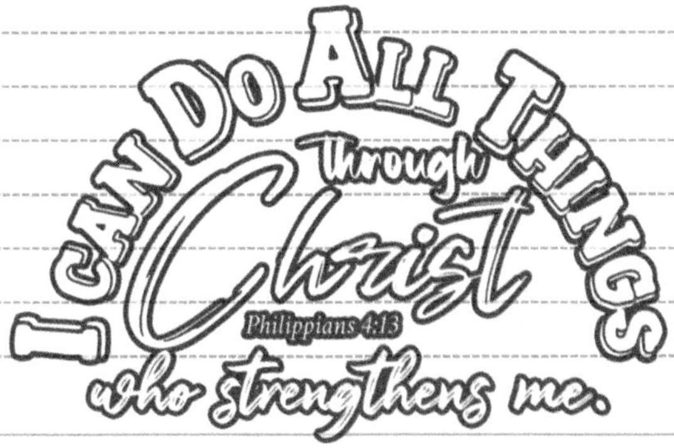
I CAN DO ALL THINGS
Through
Christ
Philippians 4:13
who strengthens me.

NOTES date ____ / ____

Count
-YOUR-
blessings

About the Author:

Dr. Painter has worked in the healthcare industry for 25 years. She holds a Bachelor's degree in Food and Nutrition/ Dietetics from Loyola University of Chicago and a Bachelor's degree in Nursing from Grand Valley State University (GVSU). In addition, she holds a Doctoral Degree in Nursing Practice from GVSU.

Her areas of expertise include food and nutrition, palliative, hospice and wound care within the adult/geriatric population. She currently works as a Certified Wound Care Specialist providing in home advanced wound care.

The recommendations provided in this book are based on clinical expertise but will not apply to everyone. Consult your health care provider regarding specific recommendations for your medical conditions and specific health care needs.

Maria A Painter, BSND, DNP, AGNP, WSOC

Made in the USA
Monee, IL
02 November 2026

67378708R00070